CONTENTS

DR. GABRIELE BURACCHI

THE ATKINS DIET

EXPLAINED EASY

WITH WEEKLY MENU' ALSO FOR VEGETARIANS AND VEGANS

Gabriele Buracchi

Nutritionist and Psychologist

WHAT IS THE ATKINS DIET?

The **Atkins diet** is a low-carb diet that is usually recommended for weight loss, or, rather, fat mass loss.

Proponents of this diet claim that you can lose weight by eating as much protein and fat as you like if you avoid foods high in carbohydrates.

Remember that **carbohydrates** are foods such as bread, pasta, sweets, but also carbonated drinks with added sugar, alcohol.

On the other hand, fruits and vegetables are also carbohydrates to all intents and purposes, even if their effect is decidedly different from what the previous carbohydrates have.

This is due to factors called **Glycemic Index** and **Glycemic Load**, which are discussed in the appropriate chapters at the end of the book.

These are easily understandable concepts that we need to know in order to carry out the diet correctly.

Since the early 2000s, many studies have shown that **low-carbs diets**, without the need to count calories, are effective for fat loss and can lead to various health improvements [1],[2].

The **Atkins diet** was originally promoted by **Dr. Robert C. Atkins**, who wrote a best-seller about it in 1972.

Since then, people all over the world have used the Atkins diet and many more books have been written about it.

The diet was initially considered unhealthy, largely due to its high saturated fat content.

Today, the effect of saturated fat on health and heart disease, in particular, is a topic of debate among researchers.

THE SATURATED FATS DEBATE

Many studies show that saturated fat consumption can increase LDL (bad) cholesterol, which is a risk factor for cardiovascular disease [3],[4].

A recent review conducted by the American Heart Association on the Impact of Saturated Fats on Heart Diseases concluded that replacing saturated fat with polyunsaturated fat can help reduce cardiovascular disease by about 30 percent --note3--.

Some reviews also suggest that replacing saturated fat in the diet with polyunsaturated fat reduces the risk of cardiovascular events, such as heart attacks and strokes [5],[6].

In the specific chapter we talk about the various types of fats to facilitate the correct choices. However, other reviews of the literature show no association between reducing saturated fat intake and reducing the risk of developing or dying from cardiovascular disease [7],[8],[9],[10].

Furthermore, some experts believe that not all saturated fats have the same effect on heart disease risk--note9--.
Others argue that diet in general is more important than identifying individual nutrients. Compared to other diets, some studies suggest that *Atkins and other low-carbs diets* may lead to greater weight loss and greater improvements in blood sugar, **HDL** (good) cholesterol, **triglycerides**, and other health markers compared to other diets. low-fat diets--note10--[11].
Whether or not low-carbs, high-fat (LCHF) diets like the Atkins diet raise **LDL** (bad) cholesterol appears to be on an individual basis.
A high fat diet for 3 weeks significantly increased **LDL** (bad) cholesterol, along with total cholesterol and **HDL** (good) cholesterol compared to the control group[12].
However, there was a large variance in individual LDL responses to the diet. Individual increases in LDL (bad) cholesterol ranged from 5 to 107%.

Another smaller study from 2021 in healthy 18- to 30-year-old women of average weight looked at the effect of an LCHF ketogenic diet on LDL (bad) cholesterol.

Eating a strict LCHF diet high in saturated fat for 4 weeks significantly increased LDL (bad) cholesterol in all study participants compared to a control diet [13].

This suggests that if you try an LCHF diet like Atkins , you should monitor your cholesterol levels to gauge your body's response.

One reason low-carbs diets can lead to weight loss is that a reduction in carbohydrates and an increase in protein intake can lead to a reduction in appetite, helping us eat fewer calories without having to think about it.

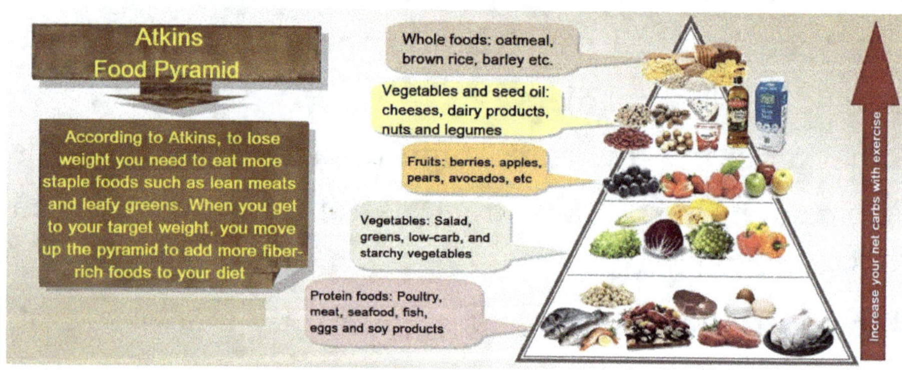

THE ATKINS DIET, A 4-STEPS PLAN

Here is a brief summary of how to follow the Atkins diet. It is always a good idea to consult your Nutritionist before starting a new weight loss diet.

The Atkins diet is divided into 4 different phases:

Phase 1 (induction): Less than 20 grams of carbohydrates per day for 2 weeks.

Therefore eat high fat, high protein, low carbohydrate vegetables such as green leafy vegetables, but also cucumbers, courgettes, radishes, broccoli, with irrelevant glycemic index.

This kicks off the weight loss.

Phase 2 (Balancing): Slowly add more nuts, low-carb vegetables, and small amounts of fruit to your diet.

Phase 3 (Fine-tuning): When you get very close to your goal weight, add more carbohydrates to your diet until weight loss slows. However, use carbohydrates with a medium-low glycemic index .

Phase 4 (Maintenance): at this point you can eat all the healthy carbohydrates that your body can tolerate without regaining weight, paying attention to those with a high glycemic index.

However, all of these steps may not be necessary. Some people choose to skip the induction phase altogether and include plenty of fruits and vegetables right from the start.

This approach can be very effective and can help you get enough nutrients and fiber.

Others prefer to stay in the induction phase indefinitely. This is also known as a low carb diet which is close to the ketogenic diet.

FOODS TO LIMIT

Individuals following the Atkins diet are told to avoid or limit the following foods: Sugar: found in sodas, juices , cakes, sweets, ice cream, biscuits and various sweets and similar products. However, sugar is a very dangerous substance for health, always.

cereals: wheat, spelt, rye, barley, rice. In any case, prefer wholemeal

"dietary" and "low-fat" foods: they are sometimes very rich in sugar.

high in carbohydrates: carrots, turnips, etc. (induction only)

high in carbohydrates: bananas, apples, oranges, pears, grapes (induction only) starches: potatoes, sweet potatoes (induction only)

legumes: lentils, beans, chickpeas, etc. (induction only)

FOODS TO EAT

While on the Atkins Diet , base your diet on the following foods:

Meats: beef, pork, lamb, chicken, bacon, and other

Fatty fishes and seafood: salmon, trout, sardines, and mackerel

Eggs: enriched with Omega-3 or pasture-raised - higher in nutrients [14][14]

Low-carb vegetables: kale, spinach, broccoli, asparagus, and other full-fat dairy products: butter, cheese, cream, full-fat yogurt

Nuts and seeds: almonds, walnuts macadamia, walnuts, sunflower seeds

Healthy fats: extra virgin olive oil, coconut oil, avocado and avocado oil.

Build your meals around a high-fat protein source with plenty of greens, nuts, and some healthy fats.

DRINKS

Here are some drinks that are acceptable on the Atkins

diet . Obviously without added sugar. **Water.** As always, water should be the drink of choice.

Coffee. Coffee, without going overboard, is rich in antioxidants and may offer health benefits. **Green tea.** Green tea is also rich in antioxidants.

You can drink alcohol in small quantities while on the Atkins diet .

Stick to dry wines with no added sugar and avoid high-carbs drinks like beer.

Obviously be careful not to overdo it so as not to frustrate the results

WHAT ABOUT VEGETARIANS?

Following a plant-based Atkins diet requires extra planning.

Because Atkins diet meals are based on high-fat protein sources (typically from meat, fatty fish, and dairy products), people on vegetarian or vegan diets need to replace them with alternatives to ensure their nutritional needs are met.

You can use soy foods for protein and eat lots of nuts and seeds. However, **olive oil** is the best source of vegetable fats.

SAMPLE ATKINS MENU FOR 1 WEEK

This is a sample menu for a week on the Atkins diet . It's suitable for the **induction phase**, but you should add more high-carb vegetables and some fruit as you move on to the other phases. **Sunday**

Breakfast: Bacon and Eggs

Lunch: Leftover Slice of Beef from the Night Before

Dinner: Grilled Turkey Breast with Gravy and Vegetables

Monday

Breakfast: Fry Vegetables and Eggs in Olive Oil

Lunch: Use the leftover stir-fry from the night before dinner

Dinner: Mackerel or other oily fish with butter and vegetables. As an alternative to mackerel, use Salmon

Tuesday

Breakfast: Bacon and Eggs

Lunch: Fish and vegetables left over from the night before

Dinner: Cheeseburger with vegetables and butter.

Wednesday

breakfast: boiled eggs with vegetables fried in butter

lunch: scampi salad with olive oil

dinner: minced chicken sautéed in a pan with vegetables

Thursday

Breakfast: omelette and vegetables, fried in olive oil

Lunch: chicken salad with oil soybeans and a handful of almonds

Dinner: Pork steak and vegetables

Friday

Breakfast: Bacon and eggs

Lunch: Chicken salad with olive oil and a handful of nuts

Dinner: Ground beef patties with vegetables

Saturday

Breakfast: Omelet with vegetables various, fried in butter

Lunch: meatballs left over from the night before

Dinner: grilled beef slice with raw vegetables, such as cucumber, tomato and garlic

Be careful to constantly vary the vegetables, raw and cooked, in your diet.

NUTRITIOUS LOW CARBOHYDRATE SNACKS

Many people find that their appetite decreases on the Atkins diet .

Some report feeling more than satisfied with three meals a day (sometimes just two).

However, if you get hungry between meals, here are some quick and healthy snacks.

a hard-boiled egg or two
a few pieces of cheese
a piece of meat
a handful of walnuts or almonds or pistachios
unsweetened full-fat greek yogurt
berries and whipped cream
baby carrots (careful during induction)
various fruits (after induction)

HOW TO FOLLOW THE ATKINS DIET WHEN EATING OUT

While it's not always the easiest way to follow the Atkins diet, many restaurants can do it.

Some tips that may help include: Ask for extra vegetables instead of bread, potatoes or rice. Order a meal of fatty meat or fatty fish.

Excellent all blue fish.

Take some extra salsa, butter, or olive oil with your meal.

A SIMPLE SHOPPING LIST

Shopping is essential. In the first place, don't go

shopping on an empty stomach and bring a list from home, buying only that.

Eating organic isn't always easy or possible, but we always try to choose the least elaborate option that fits your budget.

fatty fish: salmon, trout, mackerel and oily fish, etc.

meats: beef, chicken, lamb, pork, bacon.

prawns and shellfish .

eggs.

dairy products: greek yogurt, cream, butter, cheese.

vegetables: broccoli, garlic, cucumber, spinach, cabbage, lettuce, tomato, cauliflower, asparagus, onion, etc.

berries: raspberries, blueberries, strawberries, etc.

nuts: pistachios, almonds, macadamia nuts, walnuts, hazelnuts, etc.

seeds: sunflower seeds, pumpkin seeds, etc.

fruits: Apples, pears, oranges, watermelons, tangerines.

coconut oil and soybean oil

olives

extra virgin olive oil

dark chocolate with a high percentage of cocoa (80/90%)

avocado

Condiments: classically, sea salt is used which certainly does not add calories, but it is still advisable to use it in moderation, preferring according to taste oregano, pepper, turmeric, cinnamon, garlic, parsley, etc.

Keep in mind that many spices have a very marked therapeutic value.

RISKS

Following the Atkins diet requires you to limit some important nutrients for your body.

So, while the Atkins diet may help you lose weight and produce other favorable metabolic changes, it can also cause the following side effects, particularly early on the diet [15],[16] :

headache

dizziness

fatigue

weakness

constipation

low sugar levels in the blood

kidney problems

electrolyte imbalance.

Limiting carbohydrates in the Atkins diet also puts you at risk for insufficient fiber intake.

Fiber is protective against heart disease and some cancers, helps regulate appetite, and supports gut motility and healthy gut microbiota [17].

Much of the fiber we eat comes from whole grains and whole grain products, such as bread and pasta.

These foods are limited in the Atkins diet.

As mentioned above, the high saturated fat content of the Atkins diet can raise **LDL (bad) cholesterol** in some individuals.

This could put you at higher risk for heart disease, although research on this is conflicting.

Some research also suggests that high-fat diets, such as the Atkins diet, affect the gut microbiome .

Certain changes in the gut microbiome may be associated with an increased risk of cardiovascular disease.

A metabolite of the gut microbiota , known as a trimethylamine N-oxide (TMAO), is a predictor of incident cardiovascular disease events, such as heart attack and stroke.

In a study of the effects of several popular diets on TMAO, the Atkins diet was associated with a higher risk of cardiovascular disease (as measured by TMAO levels) than a low-fat diet [18].

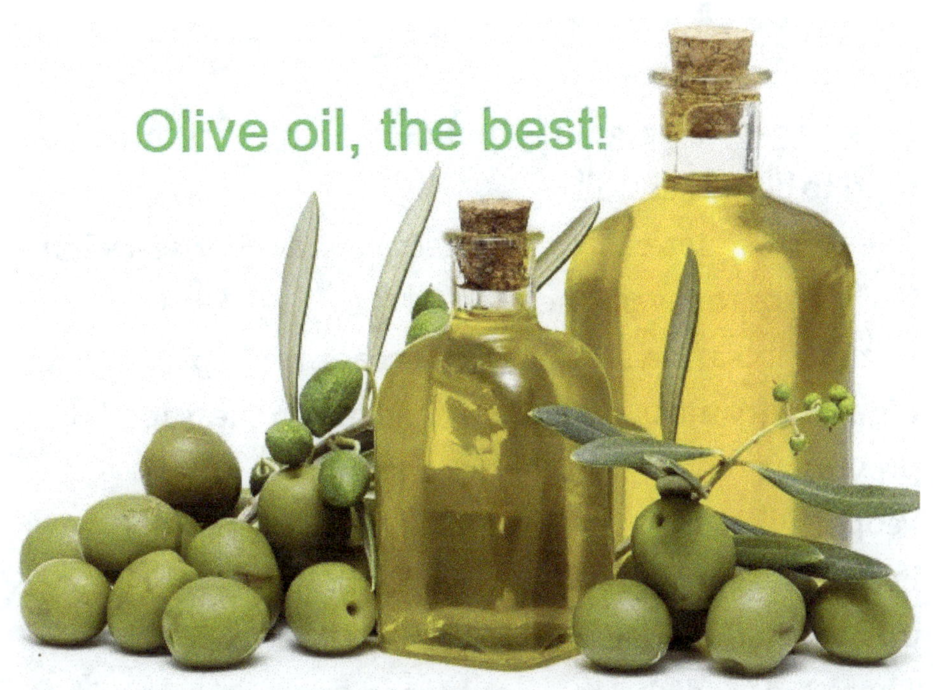

CONCLUSIONS

This step-by-step guide should contain everything you need to be successful.

The Atkins diet can be an effective way to lose weight, but it's not for everyone.

It may not always be easy to access fresh products or high quality meat, and relying heavily on these foods can prove quite costly for many people.

People with high cholesterol or an increased risk of heart disease, should monitor their cholesterol for unfavorable changes while on the Atkins diet .

Those with diabetes should consult their physician before starting the Atkins diet.

Also, people with kidney disease and people who are pregnant shouldn't follow the Atkins diet .

As always, consult a Nutritionist before starting any new weight loss diet to ensure it is suitable for your individual health needs.

JUST ONE THING

If the Atkins diet seems too limiting, but you still want

to follow a low-carb eating pattern, consider making small substitutions each week, such as replacing bread at dinner with an extra serving of vegetables or snack on veggies and nuts instead of pretzels or chips.

14 FOODS TO AVOID (OR TO LIMIT) ON A LOW CARBOHYDRATES DIET

Carbohydrates are an important source of energy and one of the three major macronutrients in the diet, along with fats and protein.

Not only do carbohydrates fuel the brain and cells throughout the body, they also regulate digestive health, appetite, cholesterol levels and more [19].

However, many people choose to limit their carbohydrate intake because low-carb diets have been linked to benefits such as greater weight loss and better blood sugar control[20].

On a low-carb diet like Atkins, you need to limit certain foods high in carbohydrates and sugar, such as sugary drinks, cakes and candies.

Yet figuring out which staple foods to avoid isn't always easy.

In fact, some high-carb foods are highly nutritious but still unsuitable for a low-carb diet.

Your total daily carbohydrate goal determines whether you should simply limit some of these foods or avoid them altogether.

Low-carb diets typically contain 20-130 grams of carbohydrates per day, depending on your goals, needs, and preferences--note10--.

Here are 14 foods to limit or avoid on a low-carb diet.

1. Bread and Grains

Bread is a staple in many cultures. It comes in various forms, including loaves, rolls, and flatbreads, or even as tortillas .

However, all of these are high in carbohydrates, whether they're made with refined flour or whole grains.

Most grain-based dishes, including rice, wheat and oats, are also high in carbohydrates and should be limited or avoided on a low-carbs diet.

While carbs' counts vary based on ingredients and serving sizes, here are the average counts for the most popular types of bread [21],[22],[23],[24]:

White bread (1 slice): 13 grams
Whole grain bread (1 slice): 14 grams
Flour tortillas (large): 35 grams
Bagel (regular): 55 grams

Depending on your carbs' limit, eating a sandwich, pizza, or chip bread can either bring you near or above your daily limit.

2. A little fruit

Eating lots of fruit and vegetables has been consistently linked to a lower risk of cancer and heart disease, also thanks to the antioxidants they contain [25],[26],[27].
However, many fruits are high in carbohydrates, so they're not suitable for a low-carbs diet.
Therefore, it is better to limit some fruits, especially very sweet or dried varieties, where the sugars are obviously much more concentrated[28],[29],[30][31].

Such as:
Apple (1 small): 23 grams
Banana (1 medium): 27 grams
Raisins (28 grams): 23 grams
Dates (2 large): 36 grams
Mango, sliced (1 cup / 165 grams): 25 grams

Berries are less sugary and higher in fibers than other fruits.
This makes berries suitable for low-carbs diets, although

people with low-carbs eating patterns may want to stick to 1/2 cup (50 grams) per day [32].

3. Starchy Vegetables

Most diets allow for an unlimited intake of vegetables. Additionally, many vegetables are very high in fiber, which can aid weight loss and support blood sugar control [33].

However, some starchy vegetables, since they contain more digestible carbohydrates and higher Glycemic Index than others richer in fiber, should be limited or avoided on a low-carbohydrates diet.

These vegetables include [34],[35],[36],[37]:
Corn (1 cup/165 grams): 24 grams
Potato (1 medium): 34 grams
Sweet potato or yam (1 medium): 27 grams
Beets , cooked (1 cup/170 grams): 17 grams.
In particular, you can enjoy plenty of low-carbs, low-GI vegetables on a low-carbs diet, including bell peppers, asparagus, and mushrooms.

4. Pasta

Although pasta is versatile and inexpensive, it is very rich in carbohydrates and above all has a medium-high Glycemic Index, which varies a little according to cooking.

Just 1 cup (150 grams) of cooked spaghetti contains 46 grams of carbohydrates, while the same amount of wholemeal pasta provides 45 grams [38],[39].

On a low-carbs diet, pasta isn't a good idea unless you're consuming a very small portion, which may not be realistic for most people.

If you really want pasta but don't want to exceed the carbohydrate limit, you can use pasta the other way around, that is, as a condiment for vegetable dishes, weighing the doses anyway.

5. Cereals

Sugary breakfast cereals are known to contain a lot of carbohydrates.

However, cereals sold for breakfast are a bad product belonging to the category of junk food, to be avoided in any case.

However, even healthy types of grains can be high in carbohydrates.

However, it is bad food for anyone, absolutely inadvisable.

For example, 1 cup (235 grams) of cooked oatmeal provides 27 grams of carbohydrates.

Steel-cut oats, which are less processed than other types of oatmeal, are also high in carbohydrates, with 28 grams of carbohydrates in each dry 1/4 cup (40 grams) serving [40],[41].

Additionally, 1 cup (110 grams) of granola offers 82 grams of carbohydrates, while the same amount of Grape Nuts (a type of packaged cereal to be avoided) contains 93 grams [42],[43].

A bowl of cereal can easily put you over your total carb limit, even before adding the milk.

6. Alcohol

Alcohol, albeit in a differentiated way, provides calories. The problem is that liquids are not as filling as solid foods and they are also foods that are very low in protein, fiber, vitamins and minerals and micronutrients in general.

Furthermore, alcohol is still dangerous to health.

Below is the calorie intake of some alcoholic beverages.

Of course, these are average values.

Spritz

This is the one that contains the least calories: about 80.

Table wine

A glass of table wine: about 87 calories.

Cognac

A shot of cognac: 90 calories.

Dry sparkling wine

A glass of dry sparkling wine: 93 calories.

Vodka

A shot of smooth vodka: 99 calories.

Sweet sparkling wine

A glass of sweet sparkling wine has 100 calories.

Champagne

A glass of champagne: 100 calories.

Grappa

A glass of grappa: 100 calories.

Whiskey

A glass of whiskey: about 110 calories. NB There are many on the market, with different strengths, some with honey: they have more calories. Bitters

A glass of amaro

about 120 calories. There are many on the market: the more sugary or alcoholic they are, the more calories they have.

Limoncello

A glass of limoncello: 130 calories.

Full-bodied red wine

A glass of full-bodied red wine: 130 calories.

Bloody Mary

A glass of Bloody Mary: 138 calories

Negroni

A glass of Negroni : 140 calories.

Cuba Libre

A glass of Cuba Libre: 150 calories.

Pint of lager

A pint of lager (40 cl): 176 calories.

Pint of stout

A pint of stout: 179 calories.

Mojito

A glass of Mojito : 200 calories.

7. YOGURT. BEWARE OF SUGAR

Yogurt is a tasty food that has many uses. Although plain yogurt is quite low in carbohydrates, many people tend to eat fruit-flavored and sweetened varieties, which often contain as many carbohydrates as dessert.

One cup (245 grams) of fat-free sweetened fruit yogurt contains up to 47 grams of carbohydrates, which is even higher than a comparable serving of ice cream [44],[45].

Instead, it's best to opt for unsweetened plain yogurt whenever possible and add your favorite low-carb toppings.

For example, 1/2 cup (125 grams) of plain Greek yogurt topped with 1/2 cup (50 grams) of raspberries keeps net carbs under 10 grams [46],[47].

8. FRUIT JUICE

Although it contains some valuable vitamins and

minerals, juice is high in carbohydrates and low in fiber, which can make it difficult to fit into a low-carbs diet.

For example, 350 mL of apple juice contains 42 grams of carbohydrates.

That's even more than the same serving of soda, which has 39 grams.

Meanwhile, grape juice contains a whopping 55 grams in the same serving [48].

Even though vegetable juice doesn't contain as many carbohydrates, a 350 mL glass still has 23 grams of carbohydrates, only 4 of which come from fibers [49].

Therefore, it would be best to control your juice intake on a low-carb diet.

9. LOW-FAT AND FAT-FREE SALAD DRESSING

You can eat a wide variety of salads on a low-carb diet. However, commercial varieties, especially low-fat and fat-free varieties, often end up adding more carbohydrates than one might expect.

For example, 2 tablespoons (30 mL) of nonfat French dressing contains 10 grams of carbohydrates while an equal serving of nonfat French dressing contains 7 grams [50].

Many people commonly use more than 2 tablespoons (30 mL), particularly on a large appetizer salad.

To keep the carbs to a minimum, dress your salad with a creamy, high-fat dressing.

Better yet, make your own homemade vinaigrette using a splash of vinegar and olive oil, which is linked to improved heart health and may support a healthy body weight [51].

10. BEANS AND LEGUMES

Beans and legumes provide many health benefits, including a reduction in inflammation and the risk of heart disease [52].

While they are high in carbohydrates, they also contain a fair amount of fiber.

Depending on your personal tolerance and daily carbohydrate allotment, it may be possible to include small amounts in a low-carbs diet.

Let's do some math on 1 cup of carbohydrates (160-200 grams) of cooked beans and legumes [53]: **Lentils**: 39 grams (23 grams net)

Peas: 25 grams (16 grams net)

Black beans: 41 grams (26 grams net)

White beans: 45 grams (30 grams net)

Chickpeas: 45 grams (32 grams net)

Red beans: 40 grams (27 grams net)

11. HONEY OR SUGAR IN ANY FORM

You probably know well that foods high in sugar, such as cookies, candies, and cakes, should be limited if you are on a low-carbs diet.

However, you may not realize that natural forms of sugar have as many carbohydrates as white sugar. In fact, many of them are even higher in carbohydrates when measured in tablespoons. Here are the carbohydrate counts for 1 tablespoon (13-21 grams) of different types of sugar: **White sugar**: 13 grams

Maple syrup: 13 grams

Agave nectar: 16 grams

Honey: 17 grams

Additionally, these sweeteners provide little to no nutritional value.

When you're limiting your carbohydrates intake, it's especially important to choose nutritious, fiber-rich sources of carbohydrates.

To sweeten foods or beverages without adding carbs, choose a low-carb sweetener instead, like Stevia .

12. CHIPS AND CRACKERS

Chips and crackers are popular snacks, but their carbs add up quickly.

These foods are also fully part of the junk food to always avoid.

Just 28 grams of tortilla chips -- or 10 to 15 medium-sized potato chips -- contains 19 grams of carbohydrates. Crackers vary in carbohydrates content, depending on how they are processed, but even whole-wheat crackers contain about 20 grams per 28 grams of product [54].

Most people eat snacks in large quantities, so they should be strictly limited if you are on a low-carb diet.

You can try making vegetarian potato chips at home or buy keto - friendly alternatives , which are usually made with ingredients like almond flour, wheat bran or flaxseed.

13. MILK

Milk is an excellent source of several nutrients, including calcium, potassium and several B vitamins.

However, it is also quite high in carbohydrates. In fact, whole milk offers the same 12-13 grams of carbohydrates per cup as low-fat and skim varieties [55].

You can add a spoon or two of milk to your coffee if you don't consume more than 3/4 a day although cream is a better option.

If you like to drink milk by the glass or use it to prepare smoothies, it is better to use almond or unsweetened coconut.

GLUTEN-FREE BAKERY PRODUCTS

Gluten is a protein found in wheat, barley and rye [56].

Some people, such as those with Celiac Disease or other gluten-related disorders, need to avoid gluten to manage digestive symptoms and prevent severe intestinal damage [57].

That said, gluten-free breads, muffins, and other baked goods aren't generally low in carbs—in fact, they often boast even more carbs than their gluten-containing counterparts.

If you're limiting your carbs intake, stick to whole foods or use almond or coconut flour to make your own low-carbs baked goods, rather than eating gluten-free processed foods.

WHY LOWERING CARBOHYDRATES MAY HELP

Although a low-carb diet is not suitable for everyone, people may choose to reduce their carbohydrate intake for many reasons.

For example, research shows that low-carbs diets can support weight loss just as effectively as other popular eating patterns, such as low-fat diets.

However, low-carbohydrate diets may have limited long-term efficacy [58].

In fact, low-carb diets such as Atkins are often recommended to treat type II diabetes, usually a consequence of eating too long a carbohydrates-rich diet.

In fact, a review of nine studies reported that a low-carbs diet helped improve long-term blood sugar control in people with type II diabetes [59].

A very low carbohydrate content as found in the ketogenic diet enables weight loss and improves insulin sensitivity, which can help improve blood sugar control [60].

Additionally, a study found that low-carbs diets may help reduce the effects of metabolic syndrome -- a group of risk factors that can increase the risk of heart disease, stroke and type II diabetes -- in people with obesity [61].

IS A LOW CARBOHYDRATES DIET HEALTHY ?

Adopting a low-carbohydrate diet (we are talking about those with a high or medium-high Glycemic Index, therefore not vegetables and only a small part of fruit) can be healthy and is linked to numerous health benefits, in particular for weight management and blood sugar control [62].

A well-planned low-carbs diet can include a variety of healthy, nutrient-dense foods, including fiber-rich fruits, vegetables, nuts, and seeds.

However, some types of low-carbs diets, such as the keto diet and Atkins, can be overly restrictive for some and unsustainable in the long run.

In my opinion, these are diets to be done for limited periods of time and only to achieve certain goals.

While the keto diet may aid short-term weight loss, it also restricts many nutrient-dense food groups and can increase the risk of some problems if followed long-term, including constipation, kidney stones, fatty liver disease, and vitamin or mineral deficiencies [63].

Additionally, very low-carbs diets may not be suitable for everyone, including children, pregnant women, and those people with certain underlying chronic health conditions, unless under medical supervision.

That's why it's best to talk to your doctor or nutritionist before drastically reducing your carbohydrate intake.

Bottom Line

When following a low-carbs diet, it's important to choose foods that are highly nutritious but low in carbohydrates.

You should minimize or avoid certain types of foods altogether.

Our choices depend in part on our health goals and personal carbohydrate tolerance.

In the meantime, focus on eating a variety of healthy foods and eating a balanced diet.

As a long-term diet, I personally recommend the Mediterranean Zone diet.

(https://www.amazon.com/dp/B0B5HP4ZSW)

10 HEALTH BENEFITS OF LOW CARBOHYDRATE AND KETOGENIC DIETS

The adoption of low carbohydrates diets has been controversial for decades.

Some people claim that these diets raise cholesterol and cause heart disease due to their high fat content.

However, in most scientific studies, low-carbs diets prove their worth as healthy and beneficial. Here are 10 proven health benefits of low-carb and ketogenic diets.

1. LOW CARBOHYDRATE DIETS REDUCE APPETITE

Hunger tends to be the worst side effect of dieting. It is one of the main reasons many people feel unhappy and eventually give up.

However, a low-carbohydrate diet leads to an automatic reduction in appetite [64].

Studies consistently show that when people cut back on carbs and eat more protein bend fat, they end up eating far fewer calories.

2. LOW CARBOHYDRATE DIETS LEAD TO INCREASED WEIGHT LOSS INITIALLY

Cutting carbohydrates is one of the simplest and most effective ways to lose weight.

Studies show us that people on low-carbs diets lose more weight, faster, than those on low-fat diets, even when the latter are actively restricting calories.

This is because low-carb diets work to flush excess water from the body, lowering insulin levels and leading to rapid weight loss in the first week or two[65].

In studies comparing low-carb and low-fat diets, people who restricted their carbohydrates sometimes lost 2-3 times more weight, without feeling hungry [66].

A study of obese adults found that a low-carb diet was particularly effective for up to six months, compared to a conventional weight-loss diet.

Subsequently, the difference in weight loss between the diets was insignificant [67].

In a year-long study of 609 overweight adults on low-fat or low-carbs diets, both groups lost similar amounts of weight [68].

3. A GREATER PERCENTAGE

OF FAT LOSS COMES FROM YOUR ABDOMINAL CAVITY

Not all fat in your body is created equal. Where fat is stored determines how it affects your health and risk for disease.

The two main types are subcutaneous fat, which is found under the skin, and visceral fat, which accumulates in the abdominal cavity and is typical of most overweight men.

The situation is different for women, in which there is also a fundamental difference between pre and post menopause.

Visceral fat tends to accumulate around the organs.

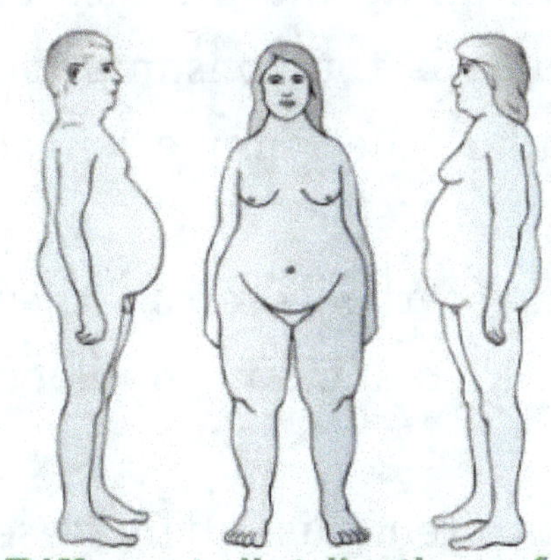

Different distribution of fat in man and woman

Excess visceral fat is associated with both inflammation and insulin resistance and may lead to the metabolic syndrome so common in the West today [69].

So low carbohydrate diets are very effective in reducing this harmful belly fat.

In fact, a greater percentage of the fat that people lose

on low-carb diets appears to come from the abdominal cavity, i.e. visceral fat, belly fat in men and post-menopausal women being the most dangerous [70].

Over time, this should lead to a dramatic reduction in the risk of heart disease and type II diabetes.

4. TRIGLYCERIDES TENDS TO DECREASE DRASTICALLY

Triglycerides are fat molecules that circulate in the bloodstream.

High fasting triglyceride levels - levels in the blood after an overnight fast - are known to be a strong risk factor for heart disease [71].

One of the main factors determining the increase of triglycerides in sedentary people is the consumption of carbohydrates, in particular the simple sugar fructose [72],[73],[74].

When people cut back on carbohydrates, they tend to experience a dramatic reduction in blood triglycerides [75],[76].

On the other hand, low-fat diets often cause an increase in triglycerides [77],[78].

5. INCREASED LEVELS OF "GOOD" HDL CHOLESTEROL

High-density lipoprotein (HDL) is often called the "good"

cholesterol.

The higher the level of HDL relative to the "*bad*" LDL, the lower the risk of heart disease [79],[80],[81]. One of the best ways to increase "*good*" HDL levels is to eat fat, especially the mono- and polyunsaturated types, and low-carb diets include a lot of fat [82] [82].

Therefore, it is not surprising that HDL levels increase markedly with healthy low-carbohydrate diets, whereas they tend to increase only moderately or even decrease with low-fat diets [83],[84].

6. REDUCING BLOOD SUGAR
AND INSULIN LEVELS

Low-carbs and ketogenic diets may also be particularly beneficial for people with diabetes and insulin resistance , which affects millions of people worldwide [85],[86].

Studies show that cutting carbohydrates, dramatically lowers blood sugar, Glicemy, and insulin levels [87],[88].

Some people with diabetes who start a low-carbs diet, may need to reduce their insulin dosage by 50% almost immediately [89][89].

In one study of people with type 2 diabetes, 95% had reduced or eliminated glucose- lowering medications within six months [90].

If you take blood sugar medications, talk to your doctor

before making changes to your carbohydrate intake, as your dosage may need to be adjusted to prevent low blood sugar.

7. MAY LOWER BLOOD PRESSURE

High blood pressure, or hypertension, is a significant risk factor for many diseases, including heart disease, stroke, and kidney failure.

Low-carb foods are an effective way to lower blood pressure, which should reduce your risk of these diseases and help you live longer [91],[92].

8. EFFECTIVE AGAINST METABOLIC SYNDROME

Metabolic syndrome is a condition highly associated with the risk of diabetes and heart disease. In fact, metabolic syndrome is a collection of symptoms, which include:

Abdominal obesity High blood pressure High fasting blood sugar High triglycerides Low levels of "good" HDL cholesterol.

However, a low-carb diet is incredibly effective at treating all five of these symptoms [93],[94].

With such a diet, these conditions are almost eliminated.

9. IMPROVED "BAD" LDL

CHOLESTEROL LEVELS

People who have high LDL *"bad"* cholesterol are much more likely to have heart attacks [95],[96].

However, particle size matters. Smaller particles are linked to a higher risk of heart disease, while larger particles are linked to a lower risk [97],[98].

Low-carbohydrates diets are found to increase the size of "bad" LDL particles while reducing the number of total LDL particles in the bloodstream [99].

Therefore, reducing your carbohydrate intake may improve heart health.

10. THERAPEUTIC EFFECT FOR DIFFERENT BRAIN DISORDERS

The brain needs glucose, as some parts of it can only burn this type of sugar.

That's why our livers makes glucose from proteins if we don't eat carbohydrates.

However, large parts of the brain can also burn ketones, which are formed during starvation or when carbohydrate intake is very low.

This is the mechanism behind the ketogenic diet, which has been used for decades to treat epilepsy in children who are unresponsive to drug treatment.

In many cases, this diet can cure children of epilepsy.

In one study, over half of children following a ketogenic

diet experienced a greater than 50% reduction in the number of seizures, while 16% became seizure free [100].

Very low-carb and ketogenic diets are also now being studied for other brain conditions, including Alzheimer's and Parkinson's disease [101].

IN SUMMARY

Few things are as well established in nutrition science as the immense health benefits of low-carbs diets.

These diets can not only improve cholesterol, blood pressure and blood sugar, but also reduce appetite, increase weight loss and lower triglycerides.

If you're curious about improving your health, one of these diets might be worth considering.

EAT LOW CARBOHYDRATES AS A VEGETARIAN OR VEGAN

Reducing carbohydrates is not very complicated. Simply replace the sugars and starches in your diet with vegetables, meat, fish, eggs, nuts and fats.

Sounds simple enough, unless you eat meat.

In fact, conventional low-carbs diets rely heavily on meat, making them unsuitable for vegetarians.

However, this is not necessarily mandatory. Anyone can follow a low-carb diet, even vegetarians and vegans.

WHY LOW - CARBS ?

Over the past 12 years, at least 23 studies have shown that low-carbs diets can help you lose weight (not counting calories).

One of the main reasons is that these diets can significantly reduce appetite, causing people to eat fewer calories without having to consciously try to eat less [102], [103].

Low-carb diets improve health in other ways as well.

They are very effective at reducing harmful belly fat and tend to reduce triglycerides and significantly increase HDL (so-called "good") cholesterol.

They also tend to lower blood pressure and blood sugar levels [104].

While low-carbs diets aren't necessary for everyone, they can have important health benefits for people with obesity, metabolic syndrome, type 2 diabetes, and some neurological disorders.

Even a low-carbs vegan diet can be very healthy.

Studies on the so-called eco- Atkins diet (vegan, 26% of calories in the form of carbohydrates) have shown that such a diet is much healthier than a normal low-fat diet, as well as a low-fat vegetarian diet [105],[106].

DIFFERENT TYPES OF VEGETARIANS

There are different types of vegetarians.

None of them eat meat or fish.

The two most common types are lacto-ovo vegetarians and vegans.

Lacto - ovo vegetarians (or simply "vegetarians") eat dairy products and eggs, but vegans don't eat foods of animal origin.

Dairy products and eggs are low in carbohydrates

Eggs and dairy products, with no added sugar, are low in carbohydrates, but high in both proteins and fats.

For vegetarians (non-vegans), they are perfect for a low-carb diet.

Eggs: contain only trace amounts of carbohydrates. Choose pasture-raised, omega-3 enriched, or free-range eggs if you can.

Yogurt, Greek yogurt, and kefir: Go for unsweetened, full-fat versions. Find those with live cultures for an added probiotic benefit .

Grass-fed: Butter from grass-fed cows is healthy and okay in moderation on a low-carb diet. **Cheese**: Highly nutritious and tasty and can be used in all kinds of recipes.

These foods are also rich in vitamin B12, which is not found in plant foods.

Vegetarians can get all the B12 they need from these foods, while vegans need to supplement.

LOW CARBOHYDRATE PLANT FOODS (FOR VEGETARIAN AND VEGAN)

There is, actually, a huge variety of low carbohydrate foods that come from plants.

Many of these foods are also high in protein and fat.

Vegetables: Many vegetables are low in carbohydrates.

This includes tomatoes, onions, cauliflower, eggplants, peppers, broccoli and Brussels sprouts. **Fruits**: Berries such as strawberries and blueberries can be eaten on a low-carb diet. Depending on how many carbohydrates you want to eat, other fruits may be acceptable as well.

Fatty Fruits: Avocados and olives are incredibly healthy. They are low in carbohydrates but high in fat.

Shell and seeds: Nuts and seeds are low in carbohydrates, but high in protein and fat.

This includes almonds, walnuts, macadamia nuts, peanuts and pumpkin seeds.

Soy: Foods like tofu and tempeh are high in protein and fat, but low in carbohydrates.

This makes them acceptable in a low-carbs vegetarian/vegan diet.

Legumes: Some legumes, including green beans, chickpeas, and others.

Healthy fats: Extra virgin olive oil, avocado oil and coconut oil.

Chia : Most of the carbohydrates in chia seeds are fiber, so nearly all of the usable calories in them come from protein and fat.

Dark Chocolate: If you choose dark chocolate with a high cocoa content (70-85%+), it will be low in carbohydrates but high in fat.

HOW MANY CARBOHYDRATES SHOULD YOU EAT?

There is no fixed definition of what exactly *"low carbs"* means. It's important to experiment and find a way to match your carbohydrates intake to your goals and preferences.

That said, I offer some guidelines, reasonable ones, obviously not of absolute value, given the differences between people: 100-150 grams per day.

This is a decent maintenance range and is good for people who exercise a lot. 50-100 grams per day: This should lead to automatic weight loss and is a good maintenance range for people who don't exercise much. 20-50 grams per day: with such a low carbohydrates intake, you should lose weight quickly without feeling overly hungry.

This range of carbohydrates should lead to ketosis.

Vegetarians could easily get into the low end, but such a diet would be impractical for vegans. The 100-150 gram range would be more suitable for vegans.

A SAMPLE MENU FOR A LOW CARBS VEGETARIAN DIET.

This is a week-long sample menu for a low-carbs vegetarian (non-vegan) diet. You can adjust it according to your needs and preferences.

Monday

Breakfast: Eggs and vegetables fried in olive oil.

Lunch: salad of four legumes with olive oil and a handful of walnuts.

Dinner: Baked Cheese Cauliflower (au gratin) with broccoli and tofu.

Tuesday

Breakfast: whole yoghurt and berries.

Lunch: Cook leftover cauliflower from the night before.

Dinner: grilled mushrooms, with buttered vegetables and avocado.

Wednesday

Breakfast: smoothie with coconut milk and blueberries.

Lunch: Carrot and cucumber sticks with hummus dip and a handful of walnuts.

Dinner: Tempeh stir-fried, with cashews and greens.

Thursday

Breakfast: omelette with vegetables, fried in olive oil.

Lunch: Stir-fried leftovers from last night's dinner.

Dinner: Chili beans with sour cream, cheese and salsa.

Friday

Breakfast: whole yogurt and berries.

Lunch: leafy greens and hard-boiled eggs with olive oil and a handful of nuts.

Dinner: Feta cheese salad with pumpkin seeds and macadamia nuts, dressed with olive oil.

Saturday

Breakfast: Fried eggs with baked beans and avocado.

Lunch: Carrot and cucumber sticks with hummus dip and a handful of walnuts.

Dinner: eggplant moussaka.

Sunday

Breakfast: Strawberry smoothie with whole yoghurt and walnuts.

Lunch: leftover moussaka from the night before.

Dinner: Asparagus, Spinach, and Feta Quiche (with or without egg).

GLYCEMIC INDEX, A FUNDAMENTAL FACTOR.

An important factor in planning and managing our diet is the **Glycemic Index.**

Whether you want to follow a low-sugar diet like the Atkins diet, or you still want to follow a balanced diet, understanding the **Glycemic Index** of foods is essential.

Why doesn't it matter what type of carbohydrate we eat? Why isn't it the same thing to eat, for example, a pound of salad and a pound of pasta?

And why is the former definitely a much better source of carbohydrates than the latter?

Apart from the enormous importance of the vitamins, antioxidants, mineral salts and fibers that salad (taken here for example from vegetables) contains and which pasta contains only insignificantly, a fundamental difference is constituted by the different speed with which these two foods cause blood sugar to rise, consequently causing a different production of insulin.

All this depends on a very important factor, the **Glycemic Index**, developed in the early 80s but unfortunately still ignored or misunderstood even by many "*experts*" in the sector.

UNDERSTAND WHAT THE GLYCEMIC INDEX (GI) IS.

Let's take into consideration a cup of sugar, a *rice cake*, some *bread*, some *cherries*, some *courgettes*, and finally a sheet of paper – perhaps the one on which your trusted nutritionist has written your diet – in any case we have taken a **CARBOHYDRATE** - or carbon hydrate or glucid or glycide, which we can also call more confidentially *sugar*.

In fact, sugars are not only those foods that appear sweet to the taste.

VARIETY OF CARBOHYDRATES IN NATURE.

There are many types of carbohydrates, or sugars, in nature.

Some, such as cellulose, pectins, hemicelluloses, as well as a wide range of gums and mucilages of various origins, are classified as fibers, i.e. they are not digestible and therefore cannot be used for energy purposes by our body.

They are only "*ballast*", but precious ballast for other functions they perform.

Yet cellulose, used to make paper, is made up of glucose

molecules just like spaghetti.

Only that the type of chemical bond with which these glucose molecules are linked together makes them unusable for us.

It's a shame, because while spaghetti also contains other substances in a small percentage, cellulose only contains glucose.

The fact is that our digestive system is not able to separate the bonds that unite these glucose molecules, something that ruminants and herbivores in general do very well.

For them, cellulose is a good food that allows them to live.

SIMPLE AND COMPLEX CARBOHYDRATES.

The carbohydrates assimilable to us are classified, from a nutritional point of view, as "*simple*" or as "*complex*".

Among the complex ones, in addition to the fibers, we remember starch, made up of linear (amylose) and branched (amylopectin) glucose polymers in variable proportions.

Simple carbohydrates, commonly called sugars, include monosaccharides such as glucose, the most common organic compound in nature - and fructose - the fruit sugar, present in many fruits and in some types of honey

-, and disaccharides, such as sucrose - the common cooking sugar extracted from beets or sugar cane -, maltose - consisting of two glucose molecules joined together through α bonds (1 → 4) and which in nature is found in discrete quantities only in sprouted seeds – and lactose – milk sugar – .

Although they are already naturally present in primary foods, sugars in refined form are used as such (sucrose) or incorporated into foods and beverages to increase their pleasantness, thanks to their sweet taste.

Until recently it was believed that the speed of absorption of carbohydrates depended on their greater or lesser complexity.

It seemed logical to assume that pasta, mainly composed of long glucose molecules joined together, required much more time to enter the circulation than, for example, fructose, the sugar extracted from fruit, which is a simple sugar.

HOW WE ASSIMILATE CARBOHYDRATES.

By checking the increase in blood sugar after ingestion of a food, however, we realized that the body follows different logics from those of some theories, logics that determine greater or lesser capacity to make us fat, but not only.

In fact, the body assimilates carbohydrates on the basis of **their Glycemic Index (GI)**, which represents the speed with which blood sugar (i.e. blood sugar) increases after consuming 50 grams of the carbohydrate in question.

Speed is expressed as a percentage by taking glucose (50 g.) as a reference point, ie by attributing it a value of 100.

This happens because the human body can only use the ingested sugars, of any type, by transforming them all into glucose.

Sometimes, especially in Italy, GI tables are found that take bread as a base 100.

In this case, just multiply the value by 0.73 to obtain the value on the glucose scale.

What do the different rates of assimilation mean.

If the food being examined has a Glycemic Index of 50, this means that the food being examined raises blood sugar with a speed equal to half that of glucose, while if it is 25, the speed will be equal to a quarter. and so on.

By going to see the GI of various foods, we thus discover some facts that were not even conceivable just a few years ago.

The same quantity of spaghetti, for example, a food considered a complex carbohydrate, can have a Glycemic Index ranging from about 35 to over 60 - it must always be remembered that glucose is worth 100 - depending on whether it is undercooked or overcooked spaghetti. Fructose, a simple sugar which, among other things, has the same calories by weight as cooking sugar, has a GI of 23, while the same cooking sugar, sucrose, in fact, has a GI of 68 , therefore not very different from that of well-cooked pasta.

The different consequences of ingesting high GI or low GI carbohydrates, regardless of whether they are simple carbohydrates or complex carbohydrates, can be seen in the graph opposite.

Why does this happen? **It's pretty simple.**

Because every time blood sugar rises quickly, the pancreas will quickly release a proportional dose of insulin, the assimilation and accumulation hormone, into the circulation.

High GI foods – as can be clearly seen by looking at the graph – will cause blood sugar to rise very quickly but, due to the effect of the insulin produced, it will quickly drop below the average level, leading to a situation of hypoglycemia.

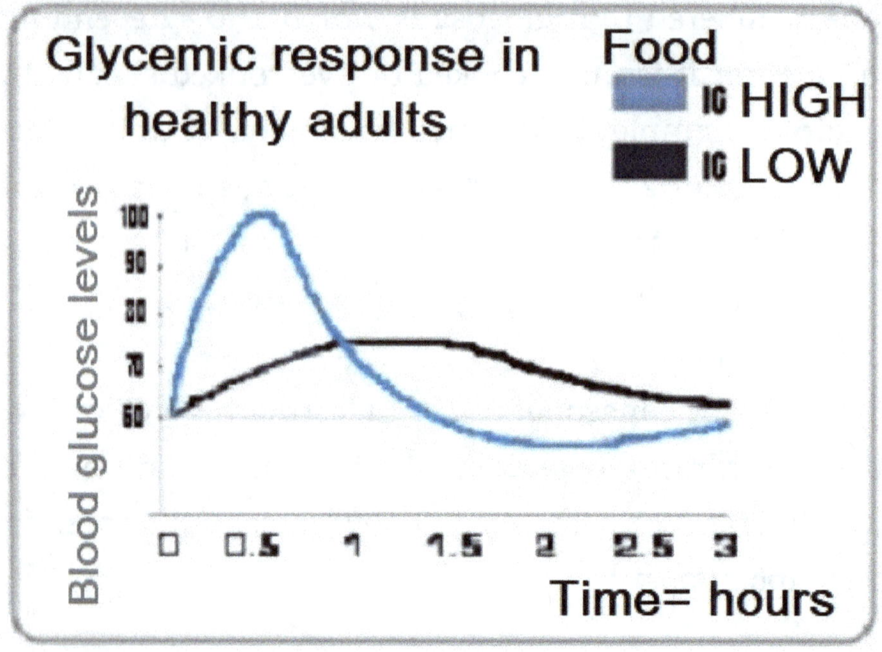

Glycemic response in healthy adults

The energy taken up very quickly will be spent by the body only in part.

When we *"fill up"* with high GI carbohydrates we cause an excessive increase in glucose - our fuel - in the blood.

Since the body is not able to tolerate hyperglycemia that much, insulin readily produced by the pancreas (under normal conditions) stores glucose in the form of fat; as a result, there will be a situation of hypoglycemia and therefore hunger, obviously for carbohydrates.

Getting fat and hungry? Basically we will end up gaining weight and being hungry at the same time.

The worst solution !

Unlike what happens with foods with a high GI, foods with a low Glycemic Index, by slowly introducing glucose into the circulation, will on the contrary allow energy to be made available gradually, giving the body time to consume it all, without accumulating a part of it as fat.

The practical consequences of what we have said are that the more we eat foods with a high GI , the easier it will be to gain weight.

So. first of all. we have to keep under control products such as sweets -obviously- but also bread, pasta, potatoes and in particular french fries but also carbonated drinks, rich in sugar and alcohol. All of these foods, including sodas, are basically all sugars and very fast sugars.

The main responsible for our fattening.

We always remember that wholemeal products have a slightly lower GI than refined equivalents, but also that a low GI product like most vegetables, if combined with a high GI product, such as pasta, reduces the risk of gaining weight-that is fat-.

Even proteins, when associated with carbohydrates, slow down their GI.

Choosing foods based on the Glycemic Index is essential!

Fats, finally, do not affect the GI in the slightest.

On the contrary, within certain limits, fats are needed in

order not to gain weight.

Therefore, instead of a plate of spaghetti without anything else, a plate of spaghetti is better, however much smaller than we are used to eating, seasoned with a little oil, with lots of vegetables and always associated with a second course.

In fact, the basis of our diet should be made up of fruit and vegetables with the right amount of protein and vegetable fats such as olive oil.

Unfortunately in our country the idea has prevailed, probably driven by interested advertisements, that the famous Mediterranean diet consists of a nice plate of pasta.

Nothing more false and dangerous. The basic foods of the Mediterranean diet are fruit, vegetables, legumes, olive oil but also fish or white meat.

And if you prefer a vegetarian diet, soy and lupine provide sufficient protein.

LOSE WEIGHT, BUT SLOWLY.

Here's the best way not to gain weight again.

It is therefore essential to lose weight only if really necessary, but above all in a slow and progressive way.

This will make it possible not to gain weight again at the end of the slimming diets, but also to avoid stretch marks and other skin blemishes that are always created in rapid slimming.

The dangers of fast weight loss diets. Losing weight with slimming diets that make you lose weight quickly is not only wrong but downright dangerous.

From what has been said on the GI Glycemic Index, consequences arise that cannot be overlooked if you really want to lose weight by avoiding the well-known Jo-Jo effect, or cyclical weight swing syndrome, as it is called in scientific jargon.

Unlike what was thought in the past – but unfortunately many continue to believe – the importance of total calories in a diet is significantly reduced.

It is not the same to assume, for example, 300 kilocalories from a low GI food such as vegetables or from a high GI food such as a dessert, but also from bread and pasta.

The value of the difference between simple and complex carbohydrates is also greatly reduced, given that the GI of a complex carbohydrate such as pasta, especially if well cooked, is very close to that of a simple carbohydrate such as table sugar -sucrose- and is much higher than that of fructose, a simple sugar extracted from fruit.

If the GI of pasta varies according to the greater or lesser cooking, so also a ripe fruit has a higher GI than an unripe fruit.

Even the GI of bread varies according to the method of production and cooking.

The Glycemic Index is also influenced by interactions with fats and proteins.

For a balanced and at the same time pleasant diet, whether you want to lose weight or want to maintain your weight, it is decidedly preferable to associate a carbohydrate-based meal – such as the classic pasta dish – with protein foods such as meat or fish or legumes, adding a certain amount of vegetable fats – olive oil – as the presence of these two macronutrients slows down the speed of intestinal absorption.

WHAT MUST NEVER BE MISSING.

Vegetables must not be missing, which with their fibers will help to modulate, reducing it, the increase in blood sugar induced by pasta.

It is therefore nutritionally more indicated to eat a plate of pasta with tomato sauce with a can of tuna rather than eating the same amount of pasta without seasonings.

And that's whether you follow a low-carb diet like Atkins or not.

Then add olive oil to the vegetables.

But for completeness it is essential to understand another concept, that of the glycemic load, which is closely connected.

GLYCEMIC LOAD.

WHAT IT SAYS MORE ABOUT THE GLYCEMIC INDEX (GI)

The effects that foods have on the body, in particular foods that act on blood sugar, depend, as already mentioned, on their Glycemic Index but also on the ingested quantities of that food.

IMPORTANCE OF AVAILABLE CARBOHYDRATES.

This means taking into account the Glycemic Load (GL), a parameter which, in addition to the Glycemic Index (GI), also depends on the quantity of Available Carbohydrates (AC) in a food.

It is intuitive that it is not the same thing, from the point of view of glycemia, to eat 50g of pasta or to eat 100, even if it is the same pasta and therefore with the same GI.

As we said when speaking of the GI , we consider sugar (meant as sucrose), rice cakes, bread, cherries, courgettes and, finally, the sheet of paper on which your nutritionist has written your diet.

FORMULA FOR THE CALCULATION OF THE GLYCEMIC LOAD.

The formula for calculating the glycemic load is: $\dfrac{GI \times AC}{100}$

Looking at the table, it becomes clear why a low-carbohydrates weight loss diet like Atkins becomes more sustainable if it is rich in fruit and vegetables.

Carbohydrate	GI	AC %	GL
sugar (sucrose)	68	100	6800/100 = 68
rice crackers	85	80	6800/100 = 68
white bread	70	56	3920/100 = 39,2
cherries	22	11,7	257,4/100 = 2,5
courgettes	15	2,3	34,5/100 = 0,3
sheet of paper	0	0	0

Values of the glycemic load of some foods

PRACTICAL EXAMPLES.

As is evident from the table, in fact, eating table sugar or the same dose of rice cakes will have the same effect on our blood sugar, and therefore on our body.

And to think that there are people who consume rice cakes believing that it is a slimming product!!!

If instead we look at the data of cherries, representative of fruit, or courgettes, representative of vegetables, we realize that their **Glycemic Load** is so low as to be practically insignificant.

This is why we can safely eat fruit and almost unlimited doses of vegetables, without consequences on blood sugar, i.e. without gaining weight.

Of course, even among fruits and vegetables there are some limited exceptions, but they are still exceptions, and in any case very relative, as in the case of bananas or carrots.

Our sheet of paper, placed there to represent nutritionally inert carbohydrates, i.e. fibers, gives a Glycemic Load of 0.

But despite this, it is strongly advised not to eat paper!!

Finally, it is useful to give just one visual example, a comparison between sugar and the most consumed food in Italy, pasta.

You probably wouldn't think so but:

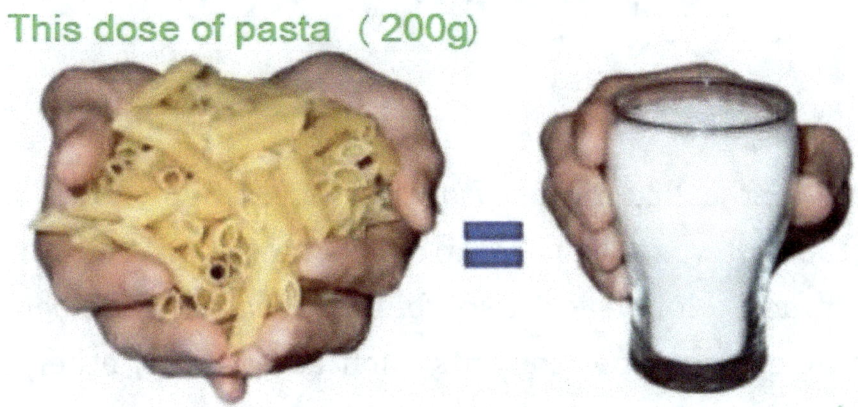

Sugar Paste Equivalence

WHAT ARE FATS

Fats, also called Lipids (from the Greek lipos = fat) are rather heterogeneous group of substances which have in common a low level of solubility in water, while being soluble in organic solvents such as benzene, ether or chloroform.

Saturated and unsaturated fat. From a chemical point of view, fats are made up of carbon, hydrogen, oxygen like carbohydrates, even if the ratio between hydrogen and oxygen is much higher.

Grasso saturo ed insaturo.

This makes them more energetic than carbohydrates in absolute terms but reduces their energy yield for the same amount of oxygen consumed.

1g of fat develops 9 K.cal against the 4 developed by a Carbohydrate.

They are found mainly in foods of animal origin (fats) but are also abundantly present in the vegetable kingdom (oils).

Even if with similar chemical structures, those that are liquid at room temperature are called oils and fats are those that are solid.

Over 500 types of fats are known which are classified according to their molecular structure as:

Simple. They are the most abundant in our body. Triglycerides, Waxes and Terpenes are simple. In our diet, about 98% of the lipids present in food are in this form.

They represent the main form of storage and use.

Composed. They are triglycerides combined with other chemicals such as phosphorus, nitrogen and sulfur.

They represent about 10% of our body's fat. Among the best known are phospholipids, glycolipids and lipoproteins.

Derivatives. They derive from the transformation of simple or compound lipids.

The most important is cholesterol, but we also remember vitamin D, steroid hormones, palmitic, oleic and linoleic acid.

Triglycerides, the simplest fats, are in turn made up of one molecule of glycerol and three of fatty acids.

Fatty Acids can be:

Saturated. So called because they have no double bonds and therefore have the maximum number of hydrogen atoms. They are found mainly in products of animal origin (eggs, milk and derivatives) but also in foods of vegetable origin (coconut and palm oil)

Unsaturated. They contain one (mono) or more (poly) double bonds between the carbon and hydrogen atoms: **Monounsaturated Fatty Acids.** They contain double bonds between the carbon atoms that compose them. They are mainly present in olive oil and dried fruit.

Polyunsaturated fatty acids. They contain more than two bonds between the carbon atoms, they are contained in fish, walnuts, sunflower oil, corn and some vegetable extracts.

For the sake of completeness, we also mention: **Hydrogenated or Trans Fatty Acids.** Normally, fatty acids of vegetable origin are liquid at room temperature. They can be made solid by the hydrogenation process which alters their chemical structure making them particularly harmful to our health.
In this way the so-called trans or hydrogenated fatty

acids are obtained, scarcely represented in nature and therefore industrially produced.

Very frequent in junk food.

Essential Fatty Acids (AGE), cannot be synthesized by the human body.

They are the precursors of prostaglandins, thromboxanes and leukotrienes , substances that intervene in the immune system, in the inflammatory response and influence the cardiovascular system.

Triglycerides are the simplest but most abundant lipids in nature.

As we have said, they derive from the union of a glycerol molecule with three fatty acids in turn formed by hydrocarbon chains ranging from a minimum of 4 to a maximum of 20 carbon atoms.

Triglycerides represent the storage form of Fatty Acids, a bit like glycogen, the storage form of glucose.

In fact, during energy processes, our body splits the bond between glycerol and fatty acids, channeling them into two completely different metabolic pathways.

While glycerol is used to produce glucose, free fatty acids are transported in the bloodstream in association with albumin, a plasma protein which transports them to the muscles where they form the energy substrate for oxidative processes.

WHO AM I

I am a Nutritionist and a Psychologist. I have worked for more than 30 years in various clinics in Tuscany in the nutrition sector, also with people with eating disorders.

I was a contract professor at the Faculty of Medicine of the University of Pisa and in others.

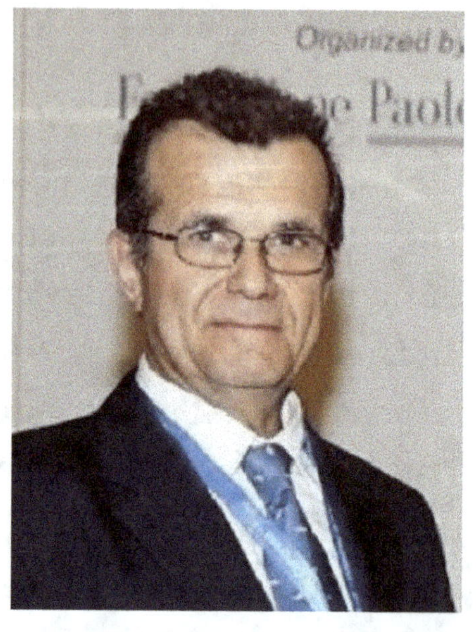

I continue to consult online through my website www.dietazonaonline.com

To find out more about me you can go to my curriculum https://dietazonaonline.com/curriculum-vitae-dott-buracchi

**If you want you can write to
g.buracchi@ gmail.com**

If you are interested in my other books on nutrition, natural health, psychology and novels, you can find me

on Amazon

https://www.amazon.it/s?k=gabriele+buracchi

some of my books on diet, nutrition and health

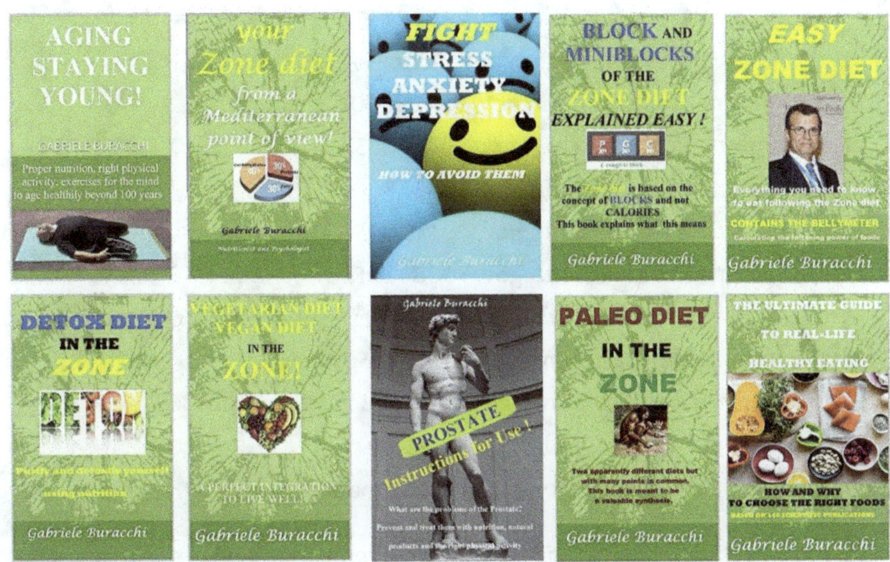

BIBLIOGRAPHY

[1] https://pubmed.ncbi.nlm.nih.gov/33441384/

[2] https://pubmed.ncbi.nlm.nih.gov/34684505/

[3] https://pubmed.ncbi.nlm.nih.gov/28620111/

[4] https://www.ncbi.nlm.nih.gov/pmc/articles/PMC7388853/

[5]] https://pubmed.ncbi.nlm.nih.gov/32428300/

[6] https://pubmed.ncbi.nlm.nih.gov/29174025/

[7] https://pubmed.ncbi.nlm.nih.gov/32428300/

[8] https://pubmed.ncbi.nlm.nih.gov/29174025/

[9] https://pubmed.ncbi.nlm.nih.gov/30084105/

[10] https://www.ncbi.nlm.nih.gov/pmc/articles/PMC6451787/

[11] https://pubmed.ncbi.nlm.nih.gov/26768850/

[12] https://pubmed.ncbi.nlm.nih.gov/30408717/

[13] [13] https://pubmed.ncbi.nlm.nih.gov/33801247/

[14] [14] https://pubs.acs.org/doi/10.1021/acsfoodscitech.0c00093

[15] Advantages and Disadvantages of the Ketogenic Diet: A Review Article - PMC (nih.gov)

[16] https://www.ncbi.nlm.nih.gov/books/NBK537084/

[17] https://pubmed.ncbi.nlm.nih.gov/33096647/

[18] https://pubmed.ncbi.nlm.nih.gov/30940489/

[19] https://pubmed.ncbi.nlm.nih.gov/29083823/

[20] https://www.ncbi.nlm.nih.gov/books/NBK537084/

[21] https://fdc.nal.usda.gov/fdc-app.html#/food-details/325871/nutrients

[22] https://fdc.nal.usda.gov/fdc-app.html#/food-details/335240/nutrients

[23] FoodData Central (usda.gov)

[24] https://fdc.nal.usda.gov/fdc-app.html#/food-details/1100713/nutrients

[25] https://pubmed.ncbi.nlm.nih.gov/27170029/

[26] https://pubmed.ncbi.nlm.nih.gov/28338764/

[27] https://pubmed.ncbi.nlm.nih.gov/28338764/

[28] https://fdc.nal.usda.gov/fdc-app.html#/food-details/1102644/nutrients

[29] https://fdc.nal.usda.gov/fdc-app.html#/food-details/173944/nutrients

[30] FoodData Central (usda.gov)

[31] https://fdc.nal.usda.gov/fdc-app.html#/food-details/169910/nutrients

[32] https://fdc.nal.usda.gov/fdc-app.html#/food-details/1102699/nutrients

[33] https://www.ncbi.nlm.nih.gov/pmc/articles/PMC7589116/

[34] https://fdc.nal.usda.gov/fdc-app.html#/food-details/1103496/nutrients

[35] https://fdc.nal.usda.gov/fdc-app.html#/food-details/170033/nutrients

[36] https://fdc.nal.usda.gov/fdc-app.html#/food-details/168484/nutrients

[37] https://fdc.nal.usda.gov/fdc-app.html#/food-details/169146/nutrients

[38] https://fdc.nal.usda.gov/fdc-app.html#/food-details/172014/nutrients

[39] https://fdc.nal.usda.gov/fdc-app.html#/food-details/168910/nutrients

[40] https://fdc.nal.usda.gov/fdc-app.html#/food-details/171662/nutrients

[41] https://fdc.nal.usda.gov/fdc-app.html#/food-details/488167/nutrients

[42] https://fdc.nal.usda.gov/fdc-app.html#/food-details/1101740/nutrients

[43] https://fdc.nal.usda.gov/fdc-app.html#/food-details/1101743/nutrients

[44] https://fdc.nal.usda.gov/fdc-app.html#/food-details/169898/nutrients

[45] https://fdc.nal.usda.gov/fdc-app.html#/food-details/1097923/nutrients

[46] https://fdc.nal.usda.gov/fdc-app.html#/food-details/1097564/nutrients

[47] https://fdc.nal.usda.gov/fdc-app.html#/food-details/1102708/nutrients

[48] https://fdc.nal.usda.gov/fdc-app.html#/food-details/1102747/nutrients

[49] https://fdc.nal.usda.gov/fdc-app.html#/food-details/1103381/nutrients

[50] https://fdc.nal.usda.gov/fdc-app.html#/food-details/1103907/nutrients

[51] https://pubmed.ncbi.nlm.nih.gov/30461730/

[52] https://pubmed.ncbi.nlm.nih.gov/26077375/

[53] https://fdc.nal.usda.gov/fdc-app.html#/food-details/175254/nutrients

[54] https://fdc.nal.usda.gov/fdc-app.html#/food-details/173143/nutrients

[55] https://fdc.nal.usda.gov/fdc-app.html#/food-details/746782/nutrients

[56] https://pubmed.ncbi.nlm.nih.gov/28244676/

[57] https://www.ncbi.nlm.nih.gov/books/NBK441900/

[58] https://pubmed.ncbi.nlm.nih.gov/33317019/

[59] Prevention and Management of Type 2 Diabetes: Dietary Components and Nutritional Strategies - PMC (nih.gov)

[60] https://www.ncbi.nlm.nih.gov/pmc/articles/PMC7480775/

[61] https://www.ncbi.nlm.nih.gov/pmc/articles/PMC6629108/

[62] https://www.ncbi.nlm.nih.gov/books/NBK537084

[63] https://pubmed.ncbi.nlm.nih.gov/29763005/

[64] https://pubmed.ncbi.nlm.nih.gov/17228046/

[65] Very-low-carbohydrate weight-loss diets revisited - PubMed (nih.gov)

[66] A Low-Carbohydrate as Compared with a Low-Fat Diet in Severe Obesity | NEJM

[67] https://pubmed.ncbi.nlm.nih.gov/12761365/

[68] https://pubmed.ncbi.nlm.nih.gov/29466592/

[69] https://onlinelibrary.wiley.com/doi/full/10.1038/oby.2006.277

[70] https://pubmed.ncbi.nlm.nih.gov/15533250/

[71] https://jamanetwork.com/journals/jama/article-abstract/207954

[72] https://pubmed.ncbi.nlm.nih.gov/11584104/

[73] https://pubmed.ncbi.nlm.nih.gov/12088525/

[74] https://pubmed.ncbi.nlm.nih.gov/23674606/

[75] https://jamanetwork.com/journals/jamainternalmedicine/fullarticle/217514

[76] https://pubmed.ncbi.nlm.nih.gov/16424116/

[77] https://pubmed.ncbi.nlm.nih.gov/1262445/

[78] https://pubmed.ncbi.nlm.nih.gov/1262445/

[79] https://www.ahajournals.org/doi/full/10.1161/01.cir.0000154555.07002.ca

[80] https://www.ahajournals.org/doi/abs/10.1161/01.cir.79.1.8

[81] https://europepmc.org/article/MED/11374850

[82] https://pubmed.ncbi.nlm.nih.gov/1386252/

[83] https://pubmed.ncbi.nlm.nih.gov/12761365/

[84] https://pubmed.ncbi.nlm.nih.gov/19439458/

[85] https://diabetesjournals.org/care/article/14/3/173/16697/Insulin-Resistance-A-Multifaceted-Syndrome

[86] https://link.springer.com/article/10.1007/s00125-002-1009-0

[87] https://nutritionandmetabolism.biomedcentral.com/articles/10.1186/1743-7075-2-34

[88] https://pubmed.ncbi.nlm.nih.gov/16403234/

[89] https://nutritionandmetabolism.biomedcentral.com/articles/10.1186/1743-7075-5-10

[90] https://www.ncbi.nlm.nih.gov/pmc/articles/PMC2633336/

[91] Short-term effects of severe dietary carbohydrate-restriction advice in Type 2 diabetes--a randomized controlled trial - PubMed (nih.gov)

[92] https://pubmed.ncbi.nlm.nih.gov/17341711/

[93] https://nutritionandmetabolism.biomedcentral.com/articles/10.1186/1743-7075-2-31

[94] https://pubmed.ncbi.nlm.nih.gov/18370662/

[95] https://www.ahajournals.org/doi/full/10.1161/01.atv.20.3.830

[96] https://www.ahajournals.org/doi/full/10.1161/01.CIR.97.18.1837

[97] https://www.ahajournals.org/doi/abs/10.1161/01.atv.12.2.187

[98] https://www.ahajournals.org/doi/full/10.1161/01.CIR.95.1.69

[99] https://pubmed.ncbi.nlm.nih.gov/16424116/

[100] https://aspenjournals.onlinelibrary.wiley.com/doi/abs/10.1177/0884533608326138

[101] https://www.ncbi.nlm.nih.gov/pmc/articles/PMC2367001/

[102] [102] https://pubmed.ncbi.nlm.nih.gov/17228046/

[103] [103] https://pubmed.ncbi.nlm.nih.gov/12679447/

[104] [104] The effect of a low-carbohydrate, ketogenic diet versus a low-glycemic index diet on glycemic control in type 2 diabetes mellitus - PubMed (nih.gov)

[105] [105] Effect of a 6-month vegan low-carbohydrate ('Eco-Atkins') diet on cardiovascular risk factors and body weight in hyperlipidaemic adults: a randomised controlled trial - PMC (nih.gov)

[106] [106]https://jamanetwork.com/journals/jamainternalmedicine/fullarticle/415074

www.ingramcontent.com/pod-product-compliance
Lightning Source LLC
Chambersburg PA
CBHW050830250726

48653CB00006B/2527